I0414243

How to Reverse Your Type 2 Diabetes

By Patricia Steele

Published by: Argon Media, LLC
1026 28th St Suite 9926
Wyoming, MI 49519

Exclusive Bonus Resource for Readers of How to Reverse Your Type 2 Diabetes

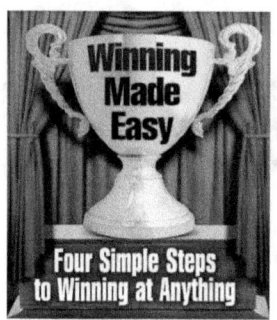

✔ Discover the 4 Steps to Winning Everyday in Every Way in your life!

✔ Learn how you can make money consistently and effortlessly.

✔ Get insider secrets to attracting and keeping your soul mate happy!

Visit http://goo.gl/sQZg9n to claim your above FREE exclusive bonus content.

Dedication
Blessed are the peacemakers, for they
Will be called children of God.   Matthew 5:9

Table of Contents

Contents

Introduction

Diabetes Mellitus is a very serious health condition. It's described as being a metabolic disease where a person's blood sugar levels are too high. This is usually because the pancreas isn't producing enough insulin to regulate blood sugar levels, or because the cells within the blood aren't responding to the amount of insulin that is being produced.

Type 2 Diabetes is the name given when the body becomes insulin resistant. This is when cells can't use the insulin the body produces properly. It's a failure within the body to respond to insulin, even though the pancreas still produces it. However, in some people there may also be a simultaneous insulin deficiency.

In 2010, there were almost 26 million American adults with diabetes. Statistics show that a further 57 million are in a pre-diabetic stage.

Pre-diabetes is the term given to people who can display some – but not all – of the diagnostic criteria for Type 2 Diabetes. This means they have an impaired level of glucose tolerance that is associated with insulin resistance. They show high blood sugar levels. It also means they're facing a massively increased risk of becoming diabetic within the near future unless they can find a way to turn those symptoms around.

Medical researchers have been keenly aware of the increasing number of people diagnosed with diabetes over the past 20 years. In fact, they now call the disease an epidemic. Dr Walter Willett published findings in the New England Journal of Medicine showing that a staggering 91% of all Type 2 diabetes cases can be prevented. Clinical studies show great success with reversing Type 2 diabetes in patients using a particular strategy consisting of diet, exercise and specific vitamin and mineral supplements.

Unfortunately, the pharmaceutical industry in America isn't interested in treating the causes of diabetes. They focus solely on treating the symptoms. The pharmaceutical industry is, after all, a multi-billion dollar industry, so it's in their best interests to continue manufacturing chemical concoctions that treat the symptoms of diabetes without actually curing it or working on ways to prevent it.

By modifying your current diet a little to include certain foods that will actively help your body to create and process insulin more efficiently and by helping to stabilize your metabolic rate, it really is possible to reverse diabetes.

If you're already taking insulin tablets or injections, it is important that you don't stop taking them right away. Instead, you need to overlap your normal doses with your natural diabetes strategies until your blood sugar levels start to stabilize on their own. At this point, you will need to work with your doctor to gradually reduce your doses so that your body doesn't suffer any adverse reactions.

Are you ready to reverse your Type 2 diabetes naturally?

Let's get started…

Why Bother Reversing Diabetes?

It's surprising just how many people are diagnosed with diabetes and have no real clue just how serious this condition is. They may understand that they require medication for the rest of their lives and they happily take that medication.

But they don't do much else to reduce or improve the symptoms of diabetes. They also don't do much about altering their current diet or exercise habits. They continue their same lifestyle, hoping the medication will fix the symptoms and nothing else needs to change.

It is true that many, many diabetics monitor what they eat and they actively cut down on sugar intake. It's also very true that many diabetic patients will try to work out ways to keep their blood sugar stable.

But these things alone won't reverse the condition. You'll still be diabetic.

Are you fully aware of the full seriousness of what having Type 2 diabetes really means? Do you know some of the major complications that arise in diabetic patients?

Let's look at some of them.

Cardiovascular Disease
All diabetics have double the risk of developing a serious cardiovascular disease. There are several major heart diseases that can develop if diabetes is left untreated, including coronary artery disease, cardiomyopathy or disease of the heart muscle, cardiac dysrhythmias or abnormal heart beat, and inflammatory heart disease.

Macrovascular Damage
Diabetics face an increased risk of damaging the large blood vessels leading to the hart, the brain and the legs. This increases the risk of heart attack and stroke enormously. Damage to the small blood vessels is also very likely, which can cause problems within the kidneys, feet and nervous system.

Stroke
As blood vessels can become damaged in diabetic patients, the risk of suffering a stroke increases dramatically.

Diabetic Coma
It's been estimated that approximately 15% of diabetic patients will experience at least one diabetic coma due to severe hypoglycemia. This is when blood sugar levels fall abnormally low, and is considered a serious complication. In some patients, seizures and even death may occur.

Diabetic Nephropathy (Kidney Disease)
Diabetic nephropathy is a progressive kidney disease, which the primary causes of chronic kidney disease and kidney failure. This is because tissue within the kidney becomes

scarred and can begin to leak plasma protein in patients where the blood sugar is poorly controlled. Treating kidney failure requires dialysis, which is an imperfect way to try and remove toxins from your blood that your kidneys should be doing for you.

Diabetic Neuropathy (Disorders of the Nervous System)
Diabetic neuropathy is a disorder that affects the major organs and peripheral nerves within your body. This can result in speech impairment, facial or eyelid drooping, incontinence or loss of bladder control, numbness within the fingers or toes, and many other symptoms besides.

Diabetic Retinopathy (Damage to the Eyes and Vision)
Damaged blood vessels within diabetic patients can lead to damage within the back of the eyes. This can result in blurred vision, development of cataracts and glaucoma, and even blindness.

Thyroid Dysfunction
While hypothyroidism is not caused by diabetes, studies do show a greatly increased risk of low thyroid levels in people with Type 2 diabetes.

Compromised Immune System
Diabetics tend to suffer from more infections than non-diabetics. This includes an increase in the number of colds, flus and pneumonia cases reported in America from diabetic patients. When blood sugar levels are high, this slows down the action of white blood cells within your body. White blood cells are designed to fight infection, so if they're compromised you're likely to be hit with more infections than you should.

Amputation
A Diabetic foot ulcer is considered a major complication of diabetes. It's estimated that 15% of all diabetics will experience this complication. It's also responsible for 85% of all foot and lower leg amputations within diabetics. As blood vessels can become damaged as a result of diabetes, this can reduce circulation within the feet and lower legs and increase the risk of developing foot ulcers and foot infections. This also reduces the body's ability to heal wounds, which can make any ulceration progressively worse. Skin and tissue may become necrotic and develop into gangrene, which also requires amputation.

When you consider just how serious the complications of Type 2 diabetes really are, it's surprising that more people don't actively search for ways to reverse the disease. Yet, it really is possible to reverse diabetes and keep your blood sugar levels under control without medication.

Are you ready to create a strategy that works for your individual lifestyle and your own body?

What's the Cause of Type 2 Diabetes?

One of the most effective ways to create a strategy to reverse a disease or condition is to first work out the most likely causes. In the case of Type 2 diabetes, there is no single contributing major cause.

However, researchers do know for certain that diet is one of the most important factors. The vast majority of Americans tend to eat a largely Westernized diet, complete with processed and pre-packaged foods. Pre-prepared foods usually contain high levels of sodium to act as a preservative. To counteract the taste of so much sodium, manufacturers add lots of sugar. Soda and alcohol contain high levels of sugar. Unfortunately, even many commercially bought fruit juices contain very high sugar content as well.

Researchers also point to being overweight as being another major contributor to becoming diabetic. Obesity has already been positively linked to insulin resistance, but even being overweight can produce the same symptoms.

Studies released by the World Health Organization and the National Health & Medical Research Council show that women with a waist measurement larger than 80cm (31.5 inches) and men with a waist measurement higher than 90cm (35.4 inches) face an increased risk of becoming diabetic. If those waist measurements increase to 90cm (35.4 inches) for women and 100cm (39.4 inches) for men the level of risk of becoming diabetic increases enormously.

The reason these particular measurements are so important is due to the way the human body stores fat. Throw out the bathroom scale immediately. You don't need it and it only serves to ruin your self-esteem anyway. Instead, grab a tape measure. This is all you need as a guide to let you know when you're on track or not.

You see, there are two different types of body fat within our bodies. These are subcutaneous fat and visceral fat. Subcutaneous fat is the layer of fatty cells right below your skin that protect your muscles, nerves and blood veins. This is the type of fat that wobbles and appears dimpled or flabby around your hips, thighs, upper arms or back.

Visceral fat is the internal fat that builds up within the abdomen to protect your inner vital organs. You can't see this on the outside on most people, except for that stubborn bloated look around your abdominal area right under your ribs and down past your belly button, but it really can do so much more damage than the layer of subcutaneous fat most people worry about.

Researchers understand that the amount of abdominal fat an obese person carries can be a very simple way to identify patients that have too much visceral adipose fat. This level of excess fat stored within the abdomen is known to cause metabolic abnormalities that slow down the metabolic rate and make it more likely that the body will become insulin resistant.

Unfortunately, when you are carrying a lot of abdominal fat it can be much harder to lose weight. This is partly because carrying fat around the middle can make your metabolism more sluggish, but also because diet alone can't shift visceral fat.

Going on a weight loss diet is excellent for reducing the amount of subcutaneous fat you have. Remember, this is the layer of fat beneath your skin that appears puffy and dimpled. Yet, visceral fat is internal. It accumulates inside your abdominal cavity and surrounds your vital organs.

The same research went further to show that people who do have excess visceral abdominal fat tend to have a very low cardio-respiratory fitness level. This is usually combined with increased insulin sensitivity and a slow metabolic rate.

When you get right down to it, Type 2 diabetes is a lifestyle disease. Eating foods that aren't right for your body's optimal health and not doing enough physical activity are the two primary causes of diabetes.

Therefore, in order to reverse diabetes you really need to stop and take a cold hard look at your current lifestyle. This is exactly how you'll work out the right strategy that will help you reverse your symptoms once and for all.

Easy Strategies for Reversing Diabetes Naturally

There are several ways to begin reversing diabetes naturally and without medication. The key to finding the right strategy to suit you is to first consider your current eating habits and your current lifestyle. Then you need to work out realistic options that work for you and your preferences.

You are an individual person with your own individual needs. Trying to create one big strategy that suits everyone is just plain dumb – and it won't work. Instead, we're going to address the three key areas that affect your body's ability to regulate your blood sugar levels and offer options you can use within your own lifestyle that work for YOU.

Now, the vast majority of tips available for trying to reverse Type 2 diabetes usually revolve around losing weight rapidly or trying to stick to unrealistic and unsustainable diets. These things sound great in theory, but they just don't work for most people.

Instead, you need to find realistic strategies that still allow you to live a normal, happy, healthy life without excessive exercise and without surgical intervention. After all, there's absolutely no point considering an extreme measure like an invasive gastric bypass surgery when you can achieve the same results naturally – and without the pain, surgery, stress and expense!

What you need to do is work on ways to incorporate some healthier choices into your current lifestyle that actually become a way of life for you without causing you undue stress. You need to work on strategies that will kick-start your metabolism so that you'll find it easier to shift that visceral fat, which will get your vital organs working more efficiently again. The result of these things combined should be that your blood sugar levels start to stabilize on their own and you become less dependent on insulin and pharmaceutical medications.

Step One: Boosting Your Metabolism

Research indicates that people with Type 2 diabetes and pre-diabetes have very sluggish metabolisms. Their bodies simply don't break down the foods they eat properly into energy, storing excess calories as fat deposits instead. Unfortunately, those people who also have a lot of visceral fat stored around the abdomen, which tends to slow down the metabolic rate even further. This actually makes losing weight even harder and makes controlling blood sugar levels difficult at best.

One of the major causes of metabolic dysfunction is a lack of water.

The second major cause of metabolic dysfunction is a lack of physical activity and poor muscle tone.

The third major cause of metabolic dysfunction is eating the wrong type of food for your body's needs in the wrong proportions at the wrong times of the day.

We're going to look at all three of these areas in some detail to show you ways to improve them without the use of strict diets and without excessive exercise. Believe it or not, there really are easy ways to address each of these areas without impacting your life too much.

Step Two: Correcting Mineral and Nutrient Deficiencies

A big problem with the Western diet is that it is deficient in many of the essential vitamins, minerals and nutrients we need in order for our bodies to function optimally. For this reason, it can be very difficult for your body to regenerate cells within your vital organs, such as your pancreas.

Taking multi-vitamins might seem like a good step in theory, but it's so important that the vitamins you take really are what your body needs. Far too many supplements available on the market are created synthetically. This means they are derived from sources grown under industrial conditions and processed using petrochemicals. This type of chemical cocktail may not be doing your health as much good as you think.

Instead, it's important to work on ways to get the essential vitamins, minerals and nutrients your body needs from as many natural sources as you possibly can. There are specific foods that can help you do this at the same time as helping to boost your metabolism.

Additionally, far too many diabetics don't eat frequently enough. When you eat two big meals through your day and skip other meals, you risk your blood sugar levels dropping too far in between those meals. When you do finally eat something, your blood sugar levels will spike making it much harder to keep them under control.

The key to reversing Type 2 diabetes through diet is to understand which foods will help you achieve your goals and which ones to avoid. You also need to understand when is the best time to eat and how big your portions need to be in order to maintain healthy blood sugar levels.

Step Three: Incidental Exercise

Almost every American is very aware that they need to get more physical activity into their day. Yet, most people have such strong negative feelings about exercise that they do nothing at all.

Let's be honest, is your first thought about exercise a picture of huffing and puffing, getting all red in the face, sweating profusely and feeling awful?

That's the image most people get when they think about exercise. What those people don't understand is that in order to achieve good health benefits and increase your metabolism, you only need to do a little in order to gain a lot.

Besides this, the visceral fat stored within your abdominal cavity that surrounds your major organs can only be reduced by physical activity. Diet won't help you get rid of this. You really do need to find some activity that helps reduce this in order to help your body function more optimally.

The key here is simplicity. A healthy amount of physical activity each day should be as natural as breathing and should be able to flow without much effort at all. You don't need to spend a fortune on gym memberships. You don't need to spend hours every day getting red in the face and sweaty. Instead, you need to work on simple, effective activities that don't require much effort at all.

When you know how, it's much easier than you think.

Once again, we'll go through this in some more detail and show you realistic, healthy ways to increase your metabolism at the same time as reducing the amount of visceral fat you store around your abdomen. The result of this will be extremely beneficial for helping your body to control and regulate your own blood sugar levels without the use of diabetic medications.

The best part about these three key steps is that they all intertwine with each other. Working on food choices and incidental exercise can be excellent for boosting your metabolism. Yet, boosting your metabolism can make incidental exercise easier for you as you should notice you have more energy during the day. Likewise, when your body is getting the right types of foods with the right amounts of nutrients, you'll boost your metabolism and find that incidental physical activity isn't a chore. So, they all serve to make every aspect of your strategy much easier on you all at the same time.

Are you ready to put these three action steps to work for your own lifestyle?

Healthy Food Choices

When most people hear the term 'healthy food choices' they immediately think of lettuce leaves and sticks of celery, which leads them to screwing their noses up at bland, boring meal choices.

Yet, there are so many ways to still enjoy all the foods you currently love without compromising on flavor.

Don't Skip Meals

It's important to keep your blood sugar levels as stable as possible when you're working to reverse diabetes. For this reason, it's equally as important that you don't skip meals.

Far too many people skip breakfast in the morning. Yet, this is the most important meal of the day. You see, while you sleep your body slows down your metabolism and uses only enough energy to keep your vital functions operating.

When you wake up in the morning, your blood sugar levels are low and your metabolism is also at its lowest point. This is why it's important you eat a healthy breakfast with at least some protein. Eggs are ideal for this. You'll kick start your metabolism for the day and help you normalize your blood sugar at the same time.

Eat Less – More Frequently

In order to begin regulating your blood sugar levels, you do need to find ways to reduce your meal portion sizes and spread the amount you eat over several meals throughout your day. This is the ideal way to keep your blood sugar levels from dipping and spiking before and after larger meals.

Vitamins and Minerals

One of the primary reasons the body starts to develop a level of insulin resistance is due to a deficiency in the vital nutrients your body needs to function optimally. Research indicates that most Type 2 diabetics have deficiencies in chromium and magnesium. Much of the food we eat is nutrient-deficient in some way, which is one reason why the multi-vitamin industry is a multi-billion dollar industry worldwide.

Choosing a good quality multi-vitamin supplement can help to restore any imbalances and deficiencies within your body. However, it's important to know which products will help improve your health and which ones are nothing more than chemical cocktails designed to part you with your hard earned cash.

Always check the labels and look for bio-available ingredients. Don't be fooled by labels that read 'whole food', as this only means that the ingredients used have been grown using bio-technology. The vitamins they want to use are then extracted using petrochemicals. This isn't natural and it's not going to help you achieve the overall healthy result you want.

Nutrient Rich Foods to Include in Your Diet

While using good quality multi-vitamins can be a great way to start addressing any nutrient deficiencies within your body, you should also look for as many ways to get those nutrients from natural sources wherever you can.

Even if you think you don't like some of the foods contained in the following list, look for recipes that sound appealing to you. Flavor your recipes with spices and herbs that appeal to your own individual taste. Look for ways to sneak little bits of vegetables into regular recipes to enhance flavor and increase your nutrient intake.

It really is easier than you think.

Here are some excellent food sources that are filled with natural, healthy amounts of vitamins, minerals and essential nutrients:

Green Leafy Vegetables
Wherever possible, try to include green leafy vegetables in your meal plans and recipes. Think about ways to include lettuce, cabbage, kale, spinach, and bok choy into recipes. Spinach is just like a vitamin pill all by itself, as it contains anti-oxidants, vitamins A, B1, B6, C, E, K, folate, chlorophyll, calcium, iron, potassium, carotenoids, potassium, protein and omega 3 fatty acids.

Fresh Fruit
Fruit does contain fructose, which leads many diabetic patients to avoid eating as much fruit as they should. Yet fruit is incredibly high in fiber. Even fruit with high fructose levels still don't cause a spike in blood sugar levels. Eat at least 2 serves of fruit each day, including apples, cherries, apricots, raspberries, strawberries, peaches, plums, blueberries, grapes, kiwi fruit, pears, bananas, mangoes, cantaloupe, watermelon, avocadoes and oranges.

Don't be fooled into thinking that fruit juices can be used as a substitute for fresh fruit. Most commercially-bought juices are processed and contain very high fructose content along with added sugar, or sweetened with high fructose corn syrup.

Beans, Peas and Legumes
Beans, peas and legumes are very high in natural fiber and they're an excellent low-fat source of protein. Add these into your meal plans whenever you can, as they're filled with B-group vitamins, along with good levels of iron, copper, folate, magnesium, potassium and lignans.

Broccoli and Cauliflower

Adding broccoli and cauliflower into your recipes can be an excellent way to increase your intake of vitamin B and C, as well as containing anti-oxidants, phosphorus, potassium, calcium, protein and chromium. These are also very high in natural fiber, so they're great for detoxifying the body.

Chili
Recipes flavored with chili can be excellent for speeding up your metabolism. This is because they produce heat within your body, which forces your body to work harder to try and cool down. Aside from this, foods within the solanaceae family like chili, capsicum, red peppers, tomatoes and eggplants contain lots of vitamin C, B-group vitamins, magnesium, iron, potassium and carotene.

Cucumber, Pumpkin and Zucchini
Any fruits within the cucurbita family are excellent additions to your meal plan. They are all high in natural fiber and very rich in vitamins and minerals, such as vitamins A, B6 and C, magnesium, calcium sulphur, silicon, potassium, niacin, thiamin, zinc, and tryptophan.

Eggs
Many diabetics struggle with high blood pressure and high cholesterol levels, so they try to avoid eating eggs. Yet, eggs offer so many nutritional benefits that it would be silly to exclude them from your diet. Besides, the American Heart Association released studies that show women who eat 2 boiled eggs for breakfast every day and who also ate a low fat diet didn't show any increase in cholesterol levels at all.

Eggs contain vitamins B2, B6 and B12, along with zinc, iron, protein, folate and lutein. When you eat the whole egg, the yolk is what contains all the vitamin A, vitamin D, vitamin E, choline, protein and omega 3 fatty acids.

Of course, if you're going to fry eggs in oil that's a whole different story. The key is to boil, poach or scramble whole eggs to get the best health benefits.

Garlic and Onion
Wherever you can, try to add a little garlic and onion into your recipes. Not only do these make great flavorings when cooked properly, but they're extremely rich in vital nutrients. Garlic can boost your metabolism by stimulating your nervous system and suppressing your appetite. Garlic is filled with vitamins A, B, C, calcium, potassium, selenium and zinc. It is also very rich in an essential amino acid called allicin, which has been proven to reduce blood pressure, reduce insulin levels and triglyceride levels.

Onions are particular high in anti-oxidants. They also contain anti-inflammatory properties and can help to reduce cholesterol, along with containing antibacterial, anti-viral, and anti-allergenic properties that are excellent for helping to boost your immune system.

Fish and Seafood
Research conducted at the Linus Pauling Institute show that a deficiency in omega 3 fatty acids can increase insulin resistance and increase blood sugar levels. In patients who increased their intake of omega 3 fatty acids, results showed a decrease in insulin resistance and improved blood sugar control.

Omega 3 fatty acids are mostly found in fish and seafood. Wherever possible, consider including tuna, salmon, sardines, trout, mackerel, oysters, prawns and other seafood into your diet a couple of times a week. Always find healthy ways to prepare and cook your fish or seafood, and avoid deep-frying it or slathering it with tartar sauce.

Chicken and Turkey

We all need a certain amount of protein in our diets in order to stay healthy. However, it's important to avoid any cuts of meat that contain high fat content. For this reason, you may want to opt for skinless chicken breast or turkey breast meat to increase your protein intake and keep your saturated fat intake down.

Foods to Avoid

There are some types of foods that can actually damage your attempts to reverse Type 2 diabetes. You may already be aware that candies and sweets really aren't going to help you to control your blood sugar levels, and you may also be trying to avoid cakes and cookies as well for the same reason.

However, there are plenty of other foods that can spike your blood sugar levels and increase the risk of diabetes complications.

These include foods such as:

- Refined sugar
- White flour
- White pasta
- White rice
- Foods containing high fructose corn syrup
- Trans fats
- Fatty cuts of meat
- Fried foods
- Soda
- Commercially-bought fruit juice
- Packaged snack foods (corn chips, potato crisps, pretzels)
- Alcohol

Dangers of MSG

Before you start thinking that MSG is no longer allowed to be used by food manufacturers in America, there is something you need to know. Mono-sodium glutamate has been positively linked to obesity in many, many studies around the world. Unfortunately, it's still used in almost every country around the world as a 'flavor enhancer'.

Because American food manufacturers are no long allowed to put MSG on food labels, they sneak it in the food anyway and disguise the name as other things. Go to your pantry right now and check out the labels on any stock cubes, soup mixes, gravy powder, packet pasta meals, instant noodles, flavored corn chips or potato crisps, or instant packet meals you have in there. Take particular notice of the labels of any 'diet' products you find. Then take a look in your freezer and read the labels on flavored ice cream and TV dinners.

You'll find MSG included in these foods, but it may be re-named as any of the following things:

- Flavor enhancer 635
- Flavor enhancer 631
- Flavor enhancer 627
- Yeast extract
- Autolyzed yeast
- Sodium caseinate
- Hydrolyzed plant (or vegetable) protein
- Corn gluten

MSG actually stimulates your pancreas, which means it tries to produce insulin in order to absorb sugar. This creates a huge insulin response after you eat it. Research conducted in Canada and published in the American Journal of Physiology shows that eating foods that contain MSG actively results in higher insulin levels within the blood.

Wherever possible, consider using fresh ingredients to make your food. Avoid processed or pre-packaged foods that may contain re-named MSG.

Boosting Your Metabolism

Increasing your metabolic rate can make it much easier for you to begin regulating your blood sugar levels. Think about this: your body needs energy for everything you do. Even involuntary functions, like breathing and digesting food and processing thoughts within your brain require energy.

Your body gets that energy from the food you eat and from fat stores within your body. When you eat too many calories throughout the day, your metabolism works hard to process them. Whatever your body doesn't need to use for fuel gets stored as more fat cells.

While there are some quick and easy things you can do to give your metabolism a temporary boost, there are some lifestyle changes you can make that will turn that boost into something more long-lasting.

Water Intake

Your body is made up of around 70% water. Yet, far too many people avoid drinking it. They reach for diet sodas, coffee, juices, or anything else they can find except plain old water.

A study conducted in the Clinical Research Center in Berlin revealed that it's possible to increase your metabolic rate by up to 30% within 10 minutes of drinking a glass of water. Aside from this, when you drink more water your body's ability to flush out excess toxins improves.

As your body becomes more hydrated, your liver and kidneys become more efficient. Well-hydrated kidneys flush toxins out of your body. A well-hydrated liver is designed to convert fat stores into energy. Without sufficient water, these vital organs can't do their jobs effectively.

Water helps your digestive system to absorb the nutrients in food more effectively. It also helps to keep your bowel functions moving properly, as a dehydrated person is more likely to have problems with constipation.

Additionally, the American Journal of Epidemiology published research that showed people who drank more than 6 glasses of water each day are 40% less likely to die of a heart attack.

If you currently don't drink enough water, you will immediately notice a side effect of drinking more. You'll end up in the bathroom a lot more frequently. Don't panic about this, as it's only a temporary side effect. This is your body's way of flushing out all the excess fluid you've been storing, so it will stop once the excess fluid is gone and you'll go back to normal.

Lean Muscle

One of the fastest ways to boost your metabolism is to work on building up lean muscle. Don't screw up your nose and imagine yourself pumping heavy weights to become a bulked-up muscle builder. That's never going to happen and it's just not necessary.

Your body is a network of muscles that require energy to operate. When you walk, your leg muscles expand and contract to propel you forward. When you sit down, your back muscles, abdominal muscles, and leg muscles operate together to get you down into a sitting position. When you lift a bag of groceries, your arm muscles are working.

These simple muscle movements require energy. That energy comes from the food you eat and from fat stores around your body. If you have good muscle tone, your body begins to burn visceral fat within your abdomen far more effectively as a fuel source.

Unfortunately, far too many overweight people have very poor muscle tone and low levels of cardiovascular fitness.

If you can find ways to improve the muscle tone within your body, you will be boosting your metabolism at the same time. Walking is the ideal way to tone leg, back and abdominal muscles. Simple isometric exercises are also easy and very effective for toning muscle quickly.

More Fiber

By increasing the amount of dietary fiber you get in your daily diet, you can effectively boost your metabolic rate. This is because your body has to work harder in order to break down high-fiber foods and then eliminate the remainder as waste. As your body works harder, it uses more energy, which in turn helps to boost your metabolism.

Research shows that the average American tends to only get somewhere between 12 and 18 grams of fiber in their daily diet. Yet, the recommended amount is supposed to be between 25 and 40 grams in order for our bodies to stay healthy.

You can increase the amount of dietary fiber you get by adding more fresh vegetables and fruits to your meals. Nuts and seeds are also excellent sources of fiber, as is oatmeal.

More Dairy Foods

Research indicates that women with a calcium deficiency tend to have a much slower metabolic rate overall. Dairy foods and vegetables rich in calcium actually help your body absorb fat more effectively.

Unfortunately, studies have also found that including lots of saturated fat may actually make insulin resistance worse. For this reason, you should aim at low fat, reduced fat or fat free dairy products wherever you can. This way you're increasing your calcium intake without increasing your saturated fat intake.

Physical Activity

Research has shown conclusively that exercise can improve insulin resistance. Back in 2008, the Center for Disease Control released guidelines that indicate we all need a minimum of 3 hours of cardiovascular exercise each week, along with 2 hours of strength training to improve muscle tone.

For any diabetic, getting enough physical activity each day is very important. Not only does simple physical activity help to boost your metabolism, it improves blood circulation, helps to improve heart health, and makes it much easier for you to control your blood sugar levels more effectively.

The biggest problem most people have is that they believe they don't have enough time in a day to do any exercise. So they do nothing.

Did you know that it only takes a few minutes every day to improve your fitness levels, tone up lean muscle throughout your body and improve your overall health as well?

It's true. Studies conducted at the University of Pittsburgh revealed that women who worked out for 10 minutes at a time at 4 different points throughout the day lost 30% more body fat than women who did a full 40 minute workout all at once.

Research conducted at the Mayo Clinic in Minnesota also shows that incidental exercise done in small increments throughout the day can have a very similar effect to working out for an hour at the gym.

This means the more frequently you do a bit of physical activity, the more you get your metabolism moving. The result of this is that you burn more fat – both visceral fat and subcutaneous fat.

It also means even small things you do throughout each day can have an incredibly helpful effect overall in improving fitness and reducing weight.

In an earlier section of this book, we discussed how important it is for a diabetic to reduce the amount of visceral fat stored within your abdomen. You can't reduce this internal fat by dieting alone. You really do need to get some physical activity into your daily routine in order to shift this once and for all.

This is where incidental exercise can be so crucial. Living a sedentary lifestyle is one of the main contributors to developing diabetes. It's also one of the primary factors for obesity.

Yet, our modern lifestyles revolve around sitting in front of the TV or computer. Working environments are also increasingly moving indoors at a desk in front of a computer. We press a button and the dishwasher does the dishes. The washing machine does the laundry. Press another button and dinner is heated up in a few minutes in the microwave.

All of these things contribute to a sedentary lifestyle that can so easily be reversed – with very little effort.

The key is to view any opportunity to be active as a bonus and not a chore.

Incidental Exercises

Simple little bits of extra activity throughout your day really do add up to a huge overall effect. Even boring chores have new meaning when you think about what they're doing to your body.

- Walking is the single most effective form of activity you can do. It's free and you learned how to do this as a toddler, so there's no training required. Take any opportunity to walk even a little extra throughout your day.

- Sweeping, mopping and vacuuming floors and rugs is activity that works your legs, arms, back and stomach.

- Pulling weeds from the garden gets you outdoors into the fresh air and burns calories. Your garden will look better too.

- Try parking the car a little further away from your destination and walking the rest of the way.

- Walk through the mall and window shop a little before going into the store. Those few extra steps get you closer to your daily total, so they all count.

- Turn on your favorite tunes while you do the dishes or laundry and dance around or wiggle it while you work.

- Fidget while you sit in front of the TV or computer. Swing your foot, wobble your knees, clench your muscles, or stretch and twist a bit while you sit. Just move around a bit instead of sitting like a couch potato.

- If you're talking on the phone, make a point of standing up or pacing around the room while you talk. Don't just sit and chat.

Toning Exercises

You really don't need to lift heavy weights in order to build lean muscle and create a toned body. In fact, it's really easy to tone using isometric exercises.

- Try squeezing just one butt cheek and then release it. Now squeeze the other. Most people find they can do one or the other, but sometimes find that one is more difficult to squeeze. This is a sign of muscle imbalance that can affect the muscles in your back and legs. Keep doing this exercise while you watch TV and you'll be toning your butt and increasing lean muscle.

- Use the same principle with toning your stomach muscles. Sit upright while you drive or watch TV or work and hold your stomach muscles in tightly for a few seconds before you release them. Do this whenever you remember and do as many as you can. You'll improve your posture and tone your stomach at the same time.

- Make a point to do some simple bicep curls with a tin of soup from the pantry every time a commercial break comes up.

- Whenever you walk, try to stand tall and hold your abdominal muscles in. This works out your abs while you walk, along with working out your leg muscles at the same time.

Always look for any chance you have to get a bit more activity into each day. All those little things you do will add up overall to helping you improve your fitness, reduce the amount of visceral and subcutaneous fat you carry, and help you reverse your diabetes once and for all.

Conclusion

Due to the fact that Type 2 diabetes really is a lifestyle disease, the only real ways to reverse it is to work on ways to change some aspects of your current lifestyle. Always be on the lookout for any opportunity to be a little more active throughout every day and think of simple things you can do to fit these into your daily routine.

Look for quick, easy recipes you can make that include healthy food options. Always look for additional ways to add nutritious foods into those recipes so that your body is getting the vitamins and minerals it needs to keep functioning optimally.

Once you start doing these small things and finding ways to incorporate them into your current lifestyle, they'll quickly become a habit. Before you know it, you'll be feeling much more energetic. You should find that your blood sugar levels don't spike so severely. Hopefully, you'll also find that it's much easier to keep your blood sugar levels regulated on your own without the help of pharmaceutical medications.

When you do turn these simple lifestyle changes into a positive habit each and every day of your life, you should be well on your way to reversing Type 2 diabetes for good.

Good luck.

Free Bonus Preview of the 15 Minute Guide to Incidental Activity

INTRODUCTION

If you really hate to exercise, you'll be very pleased to know that you can improve your fitness levels, burn fat, improve your health, tone up your body, get rid of cellulite and lose weight just with some simple incidental activity spread out through your regular daily routine.

The key to really making incidental activity work for you is to look for opportunities. Don't see moving your body as a chore. Instead, think of every opportunity as a bonus. It's just another way you get to look and feel great without going to the gym.

Start a Biggest Movers contest with yourself. To get you to think differently, researchers say we have to see a reward. So why don't you think of three things you've been wanting and give yourself a little challenge before you get it. It can be anything: a pedicure, a new fragrance, a magazine, music CD or a book. But before you buy it give yourself a milestone to hit.

If I get 3 incidental activities done today, I'll give myself _____. Just fill in the blank with your hearts desired item.

If I find 5 incidental activities today, I'll get my pedicure Friday the 14th of May at _____.
A secret to getting yourself to take action on this is to stack the odds in your favor. How? By calling, scheduling it in and living as if you've already done it.

If I complete 21 days of incidental activities, I can add $50 more dollars to my Financial Freedom Funds.

I think you get the picture. Once you own this process and make it yours you'll find yourself thinking up ways to get more rewards. This is exactly the motivation we all need and respond to since ancient days. Now, take a look at the incidental activities that work like magic.

Walking

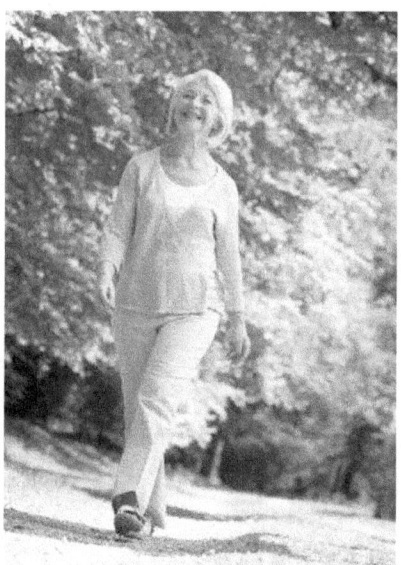

Let's be honest: not many people have the time or the inclination to walk around the neighborhood block for 30 minutes after a long day at work. This type of suggestion just doesn't work with most busy, modern families.

Instead you can use incidental activity to get your daily walking done. After all, six individual 5 minute walking sessions still adds up to 30 minutes so you're getting the same results overall.

The next time you're in the car searching for a car parking spot, don't try to circle around and look for a parking spot as close to the doors as you can find. Instead, find a park spot that is a bit further away and walk that extra minute or two to your destination. You'll find that it's always quicker and easier to find a park spot this way and you're getting those extra steps in without much effort.

Don't drop the kids off right in front of the school. Park a short distance away and walk with them. If your kids don't want you walking all the way to the school, you might want to stop a little distance away to be sure they get there before you walk back to the car.

If a friend calls you on the phone, don't drop onto the sofa to enjoy a good chat. Instead, why not pace around the room while you talk?

Always remember to stand with your back straight whenever you walk. Hold your head high and suck in your abdominal muscles as you walk. This helps to tone your stomach with every step you take and improves your posture at the same time.

Every day you should be able to find a couple of small opportunities to get even a few extra steps into your daily routine. These all accumulate to a daily total that helps you get closer to your goals.

Laughing

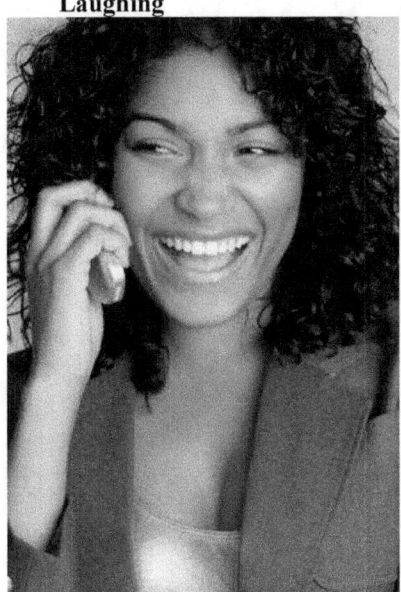

One of the easiest and most fun incidental exercises of all is laughing. Did you know that when you laugh your body is expending energy? A good old-fashioned belly laugh causes muscle contractions within your abdomen, so you're naturally using more energy to make that happen. You're also helping to tone those abdominal muscles when you really get into a good belly laugh.

Research has shown that laughing 100 times burns the same amount of energy as spending 15 minutes on an exercise bike. I don't know about you, but I'd much rather laugh my way through a silly comedy movie or hang out with friends who make me laugh than ride an exercise bike for 15 minutes!

Aside from this, when you laugh your body releases endorphins. These are your body's natural 'feel-good' chemicals. Runners get a 'runners high' because of the endorphin rush. You don't have to run, just laugh more, so you should find that you reduce stress levels naturally and you're in a better mood as a result.

Watching TV

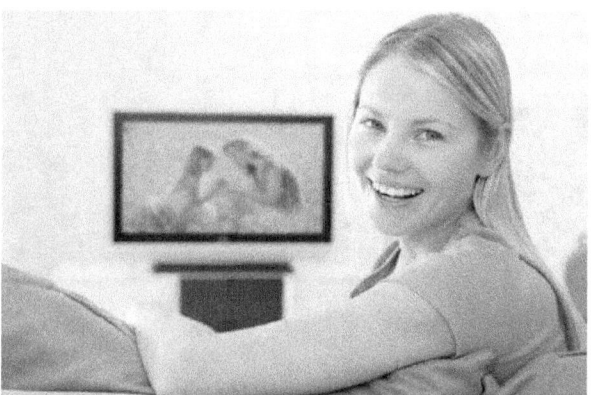

Who would have believed you can boost your fitness and tone your body while you sit on the sofa watching TV? Yet you can. The whole point of incidental exercise is to get your body moving. If you're moving, you're expending energy.

Fidget while you sit. Wobble your legs while you wait for a green light or let your foot swing back and forth while you watch your favorite show.

If you want to get a bit of body toning work done while you sit, use every commercial break as an opportunity to flatten your stomach and work on your abdominal muscles. When the ad break begins, make an effort to sit up straight in your seat. Pull your stomach muscles in tight, as though you're trying to draw them back towards your spine and hold that position for a few seconds.

This helps to strengthen your stomach and back muscles. Over time, you should notice it becomes much easier to do. You'll be improving your posture at the same time too.

Another option is to tone your butt during the break. Wait for the commercial break to start, then sit upright in your seat. Then clench your butt cheeks together tightly and hold that position for a few seconds before letting go. Repeat this activity until the ads end and your show returns. You'll be tightening and toning your butt while you sit. Terrific!

I hope you enjoy your free preview. If you'd like to read more, just buy the book where you purchased this one from.

Best wishes,
Patricia